Reiki Practices and Research

A Selective Annotated Bibliography of

Dissertations and Theses

Agnetha Leffelholz

Leffelholz, Agnetha

Reiki Practices and Research: A selective annotated bibliography of dissertations and theses/Agnetha Leffelholz

p. cm.

1. Reiki (healing system.) I. Title.

RZ 403.R45

615.8

ISBN   149965233X

ISBN-13   978-1499652338

Agnetha Leffelholz

Acupressure Practices and Research: A Selective Annotated Bibliography of Dissertations and Theses

Acupuncture Practices and Research: A Selective Annotated Bibliography of Dissertations and Theses

Reiki Practices and Research: A Selective Annotated Bibliography of Dissertations and Theses

The Sacred Feminine: A Selective Annotated Bibliography of Dissertations and Theses

All titles are also available in Large Print editions.

Table of Contents

1.)   **Barnett, D. A.**
The effects on the well-being of parents who learn and practice Reiki.
Ph.D. dissertation, Institute of Transpersonal Psychology. 2005.

Previous Reiki studies have focused on the benefits of receiving Reiki, a biofield energy medicine therapy (National Institute of Health Center for Complementary and Alternative Medicine [NCCAM], n.d.a.). This study focused on the results parents experienced by learning and practicing Reiki on themselves and their children. The hypotheses of this study was that parents who practiced Reiki on themselves and their children would experience a decrease in stress and an increase in their subjective, physical, mental, and spiritual well-being, gratitude, and family relationship quality. Participants included 48 parent volunteers experiencing stress. This study was a randomized, controlled design. Participants were randomly assigned to receive the Reiki Level One attunements or mock (limited) Reiki attunements prior to participation in a Reiki class. Participants were assessed prior to the intervention, 3 weeks after the intervention, and 6 weeks after the intervention. Assessments included the Perceived Stress Scale (PSS), Friedman Well-Being Scale (FWBS), Vitality Plus Scale (VPS), Positive States of Mind Scale (PSOM), Family Relationship Index from the Family Environment Scale (FRI), Gratitude Questionnaire-Six Item Form (GQ-6), and Spiritual Perspective Scale (SPS). For 6 weeks following their Reiki class, participants practiced Reiki or Limited (unattuned) Reiki on themselves and their children and recorded their practice time. Data were analyzed with repeated measures ANOVA, one way ANOVA, and independent and paired t tests. Results indicated that both Reiki groups experienced a statistically significant decrease in stress and an increase in well-being, family relationship quality, gratitude, and spirituality. Based on these tentative and positive results, Reiki is recommended as a transpersonal practice for self-care. However, no significant differences were found between the treatment and control group at any assessment period. Further research should investigate the mechanisms by which Reiki is hypothesized to work, such as the

attunement, simple attention, the elicitation of the

relaxation response, and/or the placebo effect.

[Author Abstract]

2.) **Caplan, L. C.**

A healing touch: Using Reiki as adjunct therapy for intractable pain.

M.S.H.S. thesis, Weill Medical College, Cornell University. 2012.

Problem: Management of intractable pain has been dominated by medication alone. With the growing prevalence of opioid abuse and dependence in the United States, it is prudent to seriously consider integrating Complementary and Alternative Medicine into pain control regimens. Reiki therapy, an energy flow therapy becoming more popular in various institutions across the country, has had scant research done exploring its efficacy. Methods: Peer reviewed articles within the last 10 years have had mixed results when measuring subjective and objective effects of Reiki. Articles were found via PubMed database using the terms "Reiki research", "Reiki" and "pain", "Reiki" and "cancer", and "intractable pain." Results: The majority of studies have found that Reiki provides a subjective decrease in pain and fatigue with a concurrent increase in energy and quality of life. However, when compared to placebo or "sham" Reiki, the studies have not been large enough or long enough to discern any significant difference from true Reiki. Conclusions: Further studies with extended courses of Reiki as compared to placebo or "sham" groups with a larger patient sample size are needed to discover if true Reiki therapy has any of the benefits practitioners claim it has, as measured both

subjectively and objectively. [Author Abstract]

3.)   **Cox, S. E.**
*Recognition, evaluation, and treatment options of
performance-related injuries in woodwind musicians.*
D.M.A. dissertation, The University of Memphis.
2009.

This document is a detailed study of the performance-related injuries experienced by woodwind musicians. Care is given to explain injuries in a language that is understandable to the non-medically trained musician. The document introduces the subject with a brief history of performing arts medicine, discussing the development and need for this highly specific specialty. This is followed by a discussion of the literature available to the musician who wants to understand performance-related injuries and how to prevent them. Chapter three is devoted to the injuries and the treatment options available to the musician. Disorders are grouped according to cause, such as overuse disorders or entrapment neuropathies, and specific anatomic locations in which the injuries are seen, such as left index finger disorders, or skin and shoulder injuries. Advice is given for discerning which injury the musician is experiencing, followed by a discussion of the typical management found in traditional medicine. Some of the causes of injuries, such as poor posture and lack of conditioning, are included. Chapter four discusses treatment of the injuries. It includes traditional medical treatment and several examples of complementary treatments that can augment or substitute for traditional medical care, depending on the musician's preferences. The complementary treatments are defined and discussed according to how they can benefit the musician. Included in this section are treatments such as massage, acupuncture, Alexander Technique, Physical Therapy, Reiki, and Reflexology. The conclusion stresses the need of all musicians for education in performance related injuries, as well as the teacher's role in recognizing and preventing these injuries. A glossary is included to explain some of the unfamiliar medical terms used to define the conditions. [Author Abstract]

4.)   **Eichhorn, T. M.**

Fragmented bodies, emerging selves: Reiki journeys and practice in south Saskatchewan.

M.A. thesis, The University of Regina (Canada). 2002.

This thesis is a study of an "alternative" healing practice called Reiki. It is the result of research conducted over the course of a year in Saskatchewan and the western United States. My participation-observation included a wide range of Reiki performances, from everyday self treatment as an initiated practitioner, to Reiki exchanges, to Reiki pilgrimage. The research also included interviews with practitioners, who interpreted experience through narrations of Reiki's central metaphor, the personal healing journey. I also draw on various sources of Reiki literature in order to compare the practitioners' interpretive narratives in everyday experience with the broader concerns of Reiki practice. To varying degrees, Reiki practitioners regard their practice as a form of resistance to conventional cultural practices in North America. A challenge to conventional medical models constitutes a small part of this effort. However, I suggest that this aspect is driven by a deeper concern; Reiki practitioners grapple with the problem of embodied personhood. This concern informs and subsumes all other in Reiki practice. In that light, I argue that though Reiki practitioners engage in an interpretive process which is predicated on the ideological assumptions of "Primitivism" (Price 1989; Slaney 1989). Through this paradigm, practitioners construct a view of the embodied person and of otherness that ultimately reinforces dominant culture. As such, I assert that Reiki is a ritual practice. Furthermore, it is a sub-cultural practice, not a paracultural or counter-cultural as some migh argue (cf. Hess 1993; Prince and Riches 1999). To the extent that it is a form of resistance, Reiki is limited by the ideology it seeks to invert and transcend. This work evaluates Dumont's schematic analysis of personhood as it compares Indian society to so-called Western society. It focuses on Dumont's discussion of relationships of encompassment, especially in terms of equality and inequality. These pertain to concepts of individualism and holism respectively..

I agree with Beteille (1986), Mines (1988, 1994), and

LiPuma (1999) that Dumont exaggerates the

homogeneity of personhood in each society and

thus denies the possibility of alternate modalities of

personhood (LiPuma 1999) in all societies.

However, I reassert Dumont's claim that

encompassment characterizes imaginings of the

person in every society. The ethnographic study of

Reiki practice suggests that notions of personhood

in the "West" are indeed predicated on the

assumption of the individual as the basis of

personhood. Alternate experiences of personhood

as holistic in Western culture are informed by

individualistic ideology. Shaped through the lens of

Primitivism they are reflections of the Western Self. Reiki is fraught with factionalism and constructions of internal otherness (cf. Hess 1993) that limit its efficacy as a form of resistance. Nonetheless, it provides a forum for practitioners to explore the potential for alternate experiences of personhood in a society that favours individualism. Without transcending its encompassing conventional paradigm, Reiki practice ritually expresses experiences in Western culture that are not typically recognized or legitimately expressed. [Author Abstract]

5.) **Ellison, R. K.**

Psi phenomena, Reiki energy healing, and spirituality within spiritual guidance: An integrative intervention model.

M.A. thesis, Institute of Transpersonal Psychology. 2012.

Psi Phenomena, Reiki Energy Healing, and Spirituality within Spiritual Guidance: An Integrative Intervention Model by Rosemary Kearney Ellison Psi Phenomena, Reiki Energy Healing, and Spirituality within Spiritual Guidance: An Integrative Intervention Model is conceived as the development of an emerging model in the practice and art of spiritual guidance. The Reiki/spiritual guidance integrative intervention is a new model that I created, and I found and elucidated the synergistic effects through this research. This thesis asks: can such an integrative effort lead one to experience a fuller sense of self as a spiritual being, providing a context for increased satisfaction and meaning, and ultimately engaging the spiritual path of one's very life? I reviewed pertinent literature to ascertain how current research illuminates the areas of influence and to identify areas for continued research to further integrate spirituality in the practice of Reiki and spiritual guidance. This research inquiry was qualitative: Methods included 2 semistructured in-depth interviews, 1 pre- and 1 post-intervention, to elicit the personal narrative of the experience of receiving Reiki/spiritual guidance. Three participants were selected from the general public, in response to the advertised Reiki/spiritual guidance research opportunity. Integral Inquiry methods included my practice of intention for the highest good and healing, ritual for the creation of safe, sacred space, and my journal observations of somatic awareness, intuitive, psychic, and synchronistic occurrences. This original research may lead to further studies that could demonstrate the efficacy and foster development of the Reiki integrative intervention as an emergent model in the practice of spiritual guidance toward wholeness--body, mind, and spirit. [Author Abstract]

6.) **Fletcher, K. S.**
Healing by touch: Energy-touch healing in the United Church of Canada.
D.Min. dissertation, St. Stephen's College (Canada). 2002.

The central topic explored in this project dissertation is the emergence and development of energy-touch healing ministries in congregational settings of The United Church of Canada. Although energy-touch healing refers to a variety of healing techniques that use the hands to transfer energy, I use the term to identify specific Christian congregational ministries that are based on Reiki, Therapeutic Touch, and/or Healing Touch. Two grounded theory research projects form the backbone of this work. The first explored how a group of United Church ministers integrated the concepts of energy-touch healing with Christian theology. The second focused on the experience of United Churches where energy-touch healing ministries have been established. In both cases, it was possible to extrapolate a theory from the experience of the participants. More specifically, a common process was employed for developing the energy-touch healing ministries in the congregations under study. The process is organic rather than linear and parallels the seasonal work of growing a garden. Certain factors that contribute to the growth of a healing ministry were isolated. These include spiritual leadership, healthy ministry relationships built on trust, and support of key members of the congregation. It was also discovered that leaders of energy-touch healing ministries draw upon similar strategies for addressing the challenges that arise as the program develops such as creating task groups to wrestle with specific issues, forming practice groups, and offering educational opportunities for practitioners and other members of the congregation. And finally, the establishment of an energy-touch ministry in the congregations under study produced a common outcome--a deepening of faith and spiritual intimacy in the participants that ultimately led to the formation of a healing community. A comprehensive description of this process is shared in the project--a guidebook titled

"Growing Energy-Touch Healing Ministries in Christian Congregations." The second project also included the development of ethical guidelines for congregations and practitioners who practise energy-touch healing in a Christian context. Both projects affirmed the social reality of healing in the particular contemporary Christian context. The stories told by the participants bear witness to the presence of healing in the lives of those who have explored energy-touch healing either as practitioners or as recipients. [Author Abstract]

7.) **Foster, D.**
The Effects of Reiki on Stress and Pain in the Hospitalized Trauma Patient.
Ph.D. dissertation, University of Maryland, Baltimore. 2010.

Stress and pain can detrimentally impact the recovery of patients in the hospital setting. Complementary and Alternative Medicine (CAM) therapies have seen an upsurge in healthcare settings. The utilization of Reiki is increasingly employed in hospitals to assist in the alleviation of stress and pain for hospitalized patients. Although progressively used with hospitalized patients, little scientific evidence as to the efficacy of this practice has been established. This study examines the effects of Reiki on both physiological measures of stress and pain (blood pressure and heart rate) and subjective measures (pain scores, amount of pain medication utilized and the State Anxiety Inventory) in hospitalized trauma patients. A quasi-experimental repeated measures study was conducted in the trauma setting. Adults (8 males and 2 females) between 23 and 59 years participated in Reiki and Standard of Care (SOC) visits on 4 consecutive days. Subjects either received Reiki or Standard of Care on day 2 and the alternate on day 3. Blood pressure and heart rate were recorded 12 times, four times during each session, with pre and post pain scores. The amount of pain medication utilized in the previous 24 hours prior to each session was recorded, as well as, the post-session State Anxiety Inventory. No significant relationship was found between age and anxiety levels (p>.05). State anxiety at the final session was found to be significantly lower than at the baseline session (p.10). No significant differences were found in heart rate and blood pressure either during sessions (p>.10) or between those receiving Reiki and those monitored for SOC (p>.10). While this study offers no support to the utilization of Reiki as an intervention for stress and pain in the hospitalized trauma patient, a discussion as to the problems and pitfalls of clinically-based research and the use of CAM is presented. [Author Abstract]

8.)   **Gibson, H. E.**
Exploring the effects of Reiki self-use on health literacy.
Ph.D. dissertation, University of Leeds (United Kingdom). 2012.

Health literacy represents the cognitive and social skills which determine the motivation and ability of individuals to gain access to, understand and use information in ways which promote and maintain good health (Nutbeam and World Health 1998:10). To date, there is a paucity of research looking at health literacy in terms of specific types of Complementary and Alternative Medicine (CAM) use. However, levels of current usage of CAM with their emphasis on raising awareness about health and healing suggest that they may be an acceptable and useful way to help

people to manage their health and wellbeing.

Reiki can be learned by anyone and, once a

person has learned it, he or she is encouraged to

regularly use Reiki on themselves as a means of

self-care. This research address the question; how

does learning and self-use of Reiki enhance health

literacy? The starting point of this multi-stage

qualitative project was the formation of a

theoretical model of Reiki health literacy based on

a critical review of the Reiki and health literacy

literature. The model was refined using

unstructured interviews with a purposive sample

of 10 Reiki Master Teachers and further explored

in semi-structured interviews with 25 Reiki level

one and two practitioners who regularly self use Reiki. Analysis of the data indicated that participants perceived Reiki as an "easy" skill to learn and valuable to use on a regular basis. Such self-use helped them make changes to their lifestyle, including diet and ways they coped at work. Reiki was used pro-actively to prevent ill-health and maintain good physical and emotional health. Participants spoke of using their Reiki knowledge and skills to self-treat minor physical ailments (headaches, muscular pains) and to manage mental and emotional problems such as worry, stress and anxiety. This research develops, refines and applies a novel model of Reiki health literacy and in doing so provides supportive evidence of the potential of learning Reiki and its regular self-use to enable a pro-active approach to health and well-being. Implications of this research include the use of Reiki as a supportive intervention for enhancing health literacy. Because anyone can learn and practise self-use of Reiki it may be a useful intervention for enhancing the health literacy skills of disadvantaged populations who are least likely to have highly developed health literacy skills. The research adds to the limited evidence base on self-use of Reiki and deepens understanding of the benefits of Reiki. [Author Abstract]

9.)   **Grant, C.**
Reiki therapy in social work practice.
M.S.W. thesis, Carleton University (Canada).
2008.

This study explores the perspectives of individuals

with Reiki and social work credentials, or

"practitioners," regarding any benefits, risks, and

barriers to the integration of Reiki therapy and

social work practice in the healthcare system. An

organizational representative from each the College

of Social Workers and Social Service Workers, The

Canadian Reiki Association, and The Ontario

Health Department was interviewed regarding

their response to the prospect of integration and for

the purpose of providing an organizational context

to the practitioners' responses. Practitioners

identified benefits to integration such as relief of physical pain, relaxation and stress reduction, relief of emotional pain, increased mental clarity and self awareness, increased receptivity to therapy, enhanced spiritual connection, and a sense of empowerment. The fit that was described between the two practices demonstrated complementary goals, values, and ethics of practice. Barriers to integration were described to be a lack of standardization in Reiki and issues around credibility, financial costs of Reiki, lack of education and scientific research about Reiki, a Western mind-set, and issues regarding touch in practice. Such barriers demonstrated the impact of cultural differences and social structures due to a conservatism around the East-West paradigm clash and the struggle to establish and maintain boundaries within both CAM groups and within the conventional medical community. None of the participants saw any risks or dangers of integrating social work and Reiki therapy. The responses of the organizational representatives demonstrated that the Canadian Reiki Association was very supportive of integration while the College and Ontario Health Department representatives took a more neutral and formalized position. These representatives cited the importance of adhering to standards of practice in their respective fields, which did not allow for an in-depth exploration of

potential issues involved with integration. [Author

Abstract]

10.)   **Hargrove, T. M.**

A phenomenological study of Reiki practitioners and their perceptions of Reiki as it relates to their personal health.

M.S. thesis, University of Montana. 2008.

The purpose of this study was to understand the essence of becoming a Reiki practitioner and Reiki's relationship to an individual's personal health. The phenomenological research perspective utilized in this study allowed the data to speak for itself and represented the essence of Reiki and Reiki practitioners in Missoula, Montana. Ten Reiki practitioners were interviewed about their personal experience with Reiki. Interviewees were all volunteers, over the age of 18, who were trained in Reiki II or higher and had more than three years of experience practicing Reiki. Participants had practiced Reiki either on themselves or someone else regularly, which was defined as at least three times per week. Collection of the data was limited to participant disclosure of the phenomena to the researcher, and by memory recall of given events. Analysis of the interview transcripts produced comprehensive data from which several themes emerged. The themes that emerged were as follows: 1) Reasons for becoming a Practitioner, 2) Balance as Health, 3) Personal Growth, 4) Facilitator & Conduit, 5) Trust & Intuition, 6) Self-care, 7) Addressing Doubts and Validation, 8) Attunements and, 9) Sensations during a Reiki Session. These themes provided a context for examining health and healing outside the biomedical model. Reiki is grounded in Chinese medicine and provides an Eastern perspective to view health and medicine. Results of this study revealed that Reiki enhances the relationship between mind, body and spirit, and initiates a redefinition of health for practitioners. Results were consistent with previous research demonstrating a relationship between Reiki and decreased stress, anxiety, and increased coping skills. Consistent with the literature, results of this study illustrated that Reiki is an effective tool for self-care and primary prevention. Reiki is a health strategy that can be invoked by anyone, anywhere at any time. Reiki would be best modeled by Health Educators as a strategy for self-care and primary prevention in conjunction with Health Behavior theories such as the Health Belief Model. It is the hope of the researcher that through the application of Reiki, the shift in Western society from secondary and tertiary prevention to primary prevention and self-care will increase. Further research is suggested in the area of Reiki and self-care and healing practice. [Author Abstract]

11.) **Hilts, F.**

An intuitive inquiry into how practitioners of spiritual
guidance and Reiki understand and experience money-
related issues in their professional and personal lives.
Ph.D. dissertation, Institute of Transpersonal
Psychology. 2010.

Money affects us at conscious and unconscious

levels throughout our lives, with heightened affects

given our current perceived negative economic

state, yet continues to be a neglected area of

research, specifically relating to interpersonal

experiences and spirituality. Twenty-five

individuals from multiple cities within the United

States who were spiritual guides and who had also

been trained as Reiki practitioners were asked to

explore their professional and personal relationship

to money. Two groups were formed based on participants' perceived relationship to money. The Pink group consisted of 13 predominantly Caucasian individuals, 11 women and 2 men, ranging in ages from 40 to 67, with an average age of 54, practicing spiritual guidance for 10 years and Reiki for over 9 years, who identified as having a positive relationship with money. The Yellow group included 12 predominantly Caucasian women, ranging in ages from 28 to 72, with an average age of 57, practicing spiritual guidance for over 16 years and Reiki for nearly 11 years, who identified as having neutral or negative relationships with money. Differences and similarities were explored between the 2 groups in the major areas of focus including how participants (a) defined money, (b) defined God and viewed the relationship between God and money, (c) felt about various aspects of their professional experience of money, and (d) personally experienced money. Ten common themes and multiple differences were identified. The Pink group defined God and money as energy. The Yellow group provided nonunified definitions for God and money. Intuitive inquiry, a qualitative, transpersonal research method was used for this study with original data gathered through interviews. This study has contributed research on money to the fields of transpersonal psychology, spiritual guidance, and Reiki, especially benefiting individuals in private practice who choose to explore professional and personal

relationships to money. [Author Abstract]

12.)	**Jankowski, J. A.**
Integrating art therapy and Reiki in treating women with addictions and trauma.
M.A. thesis, Ursuline College. 2007.

The primary focus of this case study was the integration of two expressive and holistic approaches, Art Therapy and Reiki, in the treatment of women with addictions and trauma. A selected group of seven women, residents of an adult treatment center were the participants. The main objective was to address trauma by examining the energies and various effects of trauma on the body. This was supplemented by the art therapy process. Results indicated that the participants gained numerous benefits from this combined therapeutic process. Results included: increase in relaxation, insight, self-expression, and self-esteem, while decreasing stress and anxiety. Additional research in the areas of trauma, energy work, and art therapy was recommended. [Author Abstract]

13.) **Karl, E.**
Healing from the inside out: A spiritual journey to physical healing.
Ph.D. dissertation, Union Institute and University. 2005.

This work is a multi-layered autoethnographic study of physical healing as experienced through spiritual practice. It addresses the question, "What is the mechanism behind healing?" through the academic study and experiential exploration of shamanism, Reiki and the historical Jesus. Illness and health are explored from shamanic and energetic perspectives in an attempt to see past language and discover the common experience. This exploration is accompanied by an in depth analysis of the search for the historical Jesus, in order to understand how Jesus might have developed his healing abilities. Emphasized in this project are the beliefs and spiritual practices of Jesus that may have contributed to his ability to heal. Theory is then concretized through an experiential application as the researcher utilizes a body-mind-spirit approach, documenting her own intense inner journey toward healing. The heart of this work is this personal application. The researcher recorded all elements of her internal search in a journal that became the database for the study, presented in the format of personal narrative. The process was one that utilized the mind through academic research and included the body and spirit as information learned was applied through personal spiritual practice. This process allowed the researcher to embody theory, to view it from all angles, to experience personal healing and to offer an interpretation of that healing. Concluding that this process did not enable the researcher to discover and articulate the mechanism behind healing, the researcher instead discovered that healing is a process, and revealed seven keys to healing. These are presented as suggested experiences others could pursue in search of their own wholeness. This work concludes with a metaphoric presentation of the historical Jesus as a means to frame new language around the abstract concepts involved in learning how to be a healer for self and others. [Author Abstract]

14.)   **Kelley, W. D., Jr.**

The effectiveness of Reiki as a complement to traditional mental health services.

Ph.D. dissertation, Northcentral University. 2009.

Despite its lack of mainstream support as an effective tool for helping people deal with emotional issues, Reiki treatment has been used by various practitioners that attest to its healing potential for decades. Unfortunately, very little scientific evidence exists validating the effectiveness of Reiki, and most studies that have been conducted previously have had serious design flaws or lack scientific rigor. This study looked at 73 participants in a four week treatment program for depression at a small holistic wellness center.

Participants were randomly assigned to either a control group that received traditional mental health counseling alone, or an experimental group that also received distance Reiki. Because distance Reiki was used rather than the more common hands-on Reiki, neither the clinicians nor the participants knew whether they were receiving Reiki. A quantitative experimental design was employed in which participants rated their level of depression at the start and the conclusion of treatment using the Beck Depression Index self-report form. Overall change in depressive symptoms was the dependent variable. Those receiving Reiki in addition to counseling reported a greater decrease in depressive symptoms (mean change = -18.97, SD = 14.57) as compared to those who received counseling alone (mean change = -12.61, SD = 13.27). A one-tailed independent samples t-test demonstrated that this difference was significant ($p<.05$). Although additional research with participants who were not already open to Reiki would validate this study, the findings suggest that Reiki could contribute significantly to the mental health field. [Author Abstract]

15.) **Knupp, H. M.**

Complementary and alternative medicine in occupational therapy: A survey of its use by Alberta occupational therapists.
M.Sc. thesis, University of Alberta (Canada).
2007.

This study examined Alberta Occupational Therapists' use of, and perceptions on the inclusion of eight forms of Complementary and Alternative Medicine (CAM): Acupuncture & Acupressure, Therapeutic Touch & Reiki, Reflexology & Massage, T'ai Chi, and Magnetic Therapy. The questionnaire developed was either e-mailed or mailed to all active Occupational Therapists registered with and on the contact list of the Alberta Association of Registered Occupational

Therapists (AAROT)/Alberta College of Occupational Therapists (ACOT). Total response rate was 17.14%. A total of 62 individual respondents had used CAM mostly for the treatment of symptoms. Reasons preventing CAM's use included lack of training 82.4%, interest (23%) and/or supporting evidence (22.3%). Considerations of incorporating CAM into Occupational Therapy focused on a client-centered and holistic approach to treatment (43%-63.3%), ranking above legal/employer-related aspects (43%-43.6%). Opinions on the incorporation of CAM into Occupational Therapy were generally positive, and elaborations of negative responses indicated that further supporting evidence on forms of CAM and

related research may result in changes of opinion.

[Author Abstract]

16.)   **LeBlanc, Y. L. V.**
Contemporary healing work: A social worlds analysis of Reiki in practice.
Ph.D. dissertation, McMaster University (Canada). 2010.

This dissertation examined the social history and organizational structure of Reiki (ray-key) and explored the shared ideology and intersecting involvements of fifty practitioners who are engaged in this form of energy healing work. Through a social worlds analysis I illustrate how the central process of segmentation is influencing this social world. My research reveals that Reiki is a heterogeneous set of practices with a diffuse organizational structure. Practitioners hold mixed allegiances to varying traditions and schools of practice and often develop their own unique working styles. Through their discovery of Reiki, practitioners choose to make a commitment to a twin or conjoined practice; that is, to both self healing and to the healing facilitation of others. In this dispersive and differentiated world participants developed a shared therapeutic ideology. This encompasses a core 'energetic world view' coupled with common values that include qualities of virtue, fulfillment, and respect for tacit knowledge. This therapeutic ideology buttresses personal creativity and diversity amongst practitioners. I also found that practitioners confront a continuum of public acceptance or social approval for their work that shifts from hostility to receptivity. For practitioners, although managing public acceptance was largely about defending their social world, it was also about maximizing opportunities to increase public awareness and about creating bridging opportunities that expand the boundaries of Reiki in other social world segments. This study is unique in the sociology of CAM because it offers an in-depth look at the practice of Reiki. It provides a novel sociological analysis of the processes and interactions that form, shape, and direct a contemporary healing practice. My study contributes to social worlds theory by foregrounding the salience of the actions, interactions, and experiences of front-line practitioners engaged in this community of practice. [Author Abstract]

17.)   **Lin, B.**

*The connective energetic web: Healing and ecological
awareness through Reiki.*

M.A. thesis, Royal Roads University (Canada).
2010.

Reiki philosophy and practice encourages self-
awareness, mindfulness and responsibility, which
offer unique opportunities in developing
environmentally conscious people. Various
environmental thinkers and environmental
educators have associated the environmental crisis
to the fragmentation of our society. They believe
this has led humans to become disconnected from
the environment (Capra, 1996; Berry, 1988; Fox,
1999; Macy, 2007; Lipton & Bhaerman, 2009). This
research explores the possibility of using Reiki to

reconnect people to the environment and foster the development of ecologically conscious people. The study examines the environmental and ecological principles taught by Reiki masters in their classrooms. The phenomenological approach was used as a framework to understand and describe the lived experiences of five Reiki master participants (co-researchers). In-depth interviews were transcribed for thematic analysis. Reiki is a form of transformative education which can supplement existing environmental education and integrate healing, spirituality, and environmental education. [Author Abstract]

18.)   **Macpherson, J. A.**
Gender, Reiki and energetic healing: an exploration of holistic / 'New Age' healing in Scotland.
Ph.D. dissertation, University of Stirling (United Kingdom). 2004.

Within, this thesis I provide the first empirical academic study of energetic healing, Reiki and dowsing in central Scotland, with the focus of my research being on the teaching of energetic healing in workshops (the Salisbury and Westbank centres being key locations) and related textual material. This thesis is also a step towards addressing the historical imbalance of writing about New Age beliefs and practices from a predominantly androcentric positioning, as I place emphasis on exploring how gendered spiritualities may be actively constructed in this setting. For as Dominic Corrywright has stated "the web of New Age spiritualities is crucially sustained by the individual and collective weavings of women and this is particularly evident in healing and therapies" (2003: 131). I argue that women's predominance in healing circles has a lot to do with personal projects of redefinition and self-transformation. This sort of 'work on the self does not occur under, as radical feminists Daly (1991) and Sjoo (1994) would state, overarching patriarchal paradigms. Rather 'healing of the self' is located within fluid "fields of force" (Foucault, 1980). Therefore throughout this thesis I build up a decentralised narrative of power and locate women as active healing agents. In order to construct this narrative I draw from research in the fields of Goddess and women's spiritualities, for here we find useful evaluations of how women re-inscribe their bodies as sacred and empowered through, in the former, imminent ties to the Goddess. I relate my research to Meredith McGuire's empirical study of healing in the American context, where she argues that "If the creation, maintenance and transformation of individuals gender identities are indeed among the foremost identity work to be accomplished, then extensive empirical study of the many contemporary instances of gendered spirituality is very worthwhile" (McGuire, 1994: 254). Hence in the first two chapters of this thesis I engage with feminist and ethnographic theory in general. I argue that discourses of power are multivalent operating within academic, religious, bio-medical and holistic healing circles and at the individual level. For debates abound in relation to, for example, the prioritisation of text over experiential practice - the latter being central to New Age healing in Scotland. I introduce my location as a bothsider, an academic researcher and a practising healer as this positioning has raised its own particular set of theoretical and personal questions. And I draw in the aforementioned research in the parallel fields of Goddess and women's spiritualities. Chapter three engages with representations of "the body as energetic" at the micro 'in the field' level and is primarily descriptive. Within these pages I provide a picture of how the energetic body is discursively constructed hence providing some necessary background for later ethnographic material. In chapter four I also build on the previous chapter in relation to healing and curing models of health. I adopt Meredith McGuire's analytical framework of healing types. In this way I can locate my narrative of women's power and consciousness of healing into the debates between male dominated biomedical approaches to health and the apparently more egalitarian holistic (mind, body and spirit) approaches to the same. Chapters five and six focus specifically on the healing practice and discourses of Reiki, this healing modality growing significantly in popularity in Scotland. I will propose that Reiki provides the practitioner with contrasting notions of "the healthy body" to biomedical and mainstream religious significations of the same and enables the development of empowered models of subjectivity "as healer". The technique of dowsing, which is explored in chapter seven, is regarded in healing circles as being a "visible expression" of intuitive practice. Hence learning to dowse appears to provide additional confirmation for women healers of their ability to work as more autonomous agents. For dowsing practice falls within the umbrella of earth mysteries or Gaian traditions, where the earth is seen to be a conscious, living, self-regulating entity and is identified with as the "Goddess imminent". In the final chapter I pull this thesis together as a whole and return to some of the questions asked in my opening material, noting my distinctive contributions to healing research as "a bothsider". Throughout I acknowledge that my location as 'researcher/healer' is just as materially and politically located as are healers in the field. For I, as well as 'the subjects under study', operate within fluid fields of force. Overall, I place emphasis on evaluating distributions of power and the development of new liberating models of subjectivity in healing epistemologies. [Author Abstract]

19.) **Magnuson, M. J.**

The experience and benefits of Reiki as a complement to group therapy for mothers healing from child sexual abuse.

M.S.W. thesis, The University of Regina (Canada). 2003.

This research study was designed to uncover the experience and benefits of Reiki, a holistic spiritual touch therapy, when used as a complement to traditional group therapy for Mothers healing from the impact of child sexual abuse (CSA). Traumatic memory from CSA gets lodged in cellular tissue producing symptoms of Complex Post Traumatic Stress Disorder (PTSD). Conventional treatments fall short the recognition and treatment of CSA. Recent research suggests that Reiki healing reduces symptoms of Complex PTSD. These therapies are generally not offered through public human service delivery systems such as healthcare. This study researched two groups of survivors of CSA. The first group, referred to as the Mothers' Group, added Reiki healing and Reiki Level I training to group talk therapy. In the Reiki Exchange Group, graduates from a previous Mothers' Group continued to practice Reiki and acquired Level II Reiki training. Multiple in-depth interviews uncovered the symptoms and context of CSA, as well as the participants' perceptions of the experience and benefits of Reiki. A thematic analysis revealed that Reiki training and healing reduced symptoms of trauma, improved parent-child relationships, increased confidence and responsibility in self-healing, and the increased spirituality. The reduction in anxiety was triangulated through the State-Trait Anxiety Inventory (STAI). Further benefits appeared in the formation of a collective healing environment that transformed individual responsibility for health into a mutual effort, with participants healing family, community members, and each other. The results indicate that Reiki, when combined with traditional approaches to healing, is cost-effective, empowering, and heals survivors from trauma more effectively than talk therapy alone. Healing from CSA requires holistic and multidisciplinary care that involves both professional and community expertise. The healing hands of Reiki can be taught and used as a lay therapy in various community and professional settings for the prevention and treatment of chronic health conditions. The utilization of Reiki healing can result in increased responsibility and resilience in population health, and a cost-reduction to our health and social service systems. [Author Abstract]

20.) **Markides, E. J.**

Complementary energetic practices: An exploration into the world of Maine women healers.

Ed.D. dissertation, The University of Maine. 1996.

Over the last decade a major change has occurred in the U.S. health care model for human development and health services. As early as 1947, the World Health Organization defined health as "physical, mental, and social well-being, not merely the absence of disease or infirmity. Recently "spiritual well-being" was added to this definition. This shift from an illness or remediation towards a wellness model offered the profession of counselor education an opportunity to differentiate itself from all other mental health disciplines and ground itself in an educational orientation. Building on this philosophical shift this study employed a phenomenological perspective that explored, through thematic analysis, the structure of the lived experience of twenty-four women healers in the state of Maine. This perspective combined a focus on the overall meaning of the healing practices being investigated with an emphasis on selected passages in the interviews that illustrated important themes of complementary energetic practices. Complementary practices refer to the wide range of modalities that fall outside the established fields of the medical and mental health professions. Specific practices explored in this study were: acupuncture, craniosacral therapy, emotional cleansing work, direct energy work, homeopathy, osteopathic medicine, polarity therapy, Qigong, Reiki, therapeutic touch, and vibrational medicine. Based on their state-wide reputation, two women healers were selected to represent each of the eleven modalities covered in this study to permit both within-group as well as between-group comparisons. Two traditional medical doctors were also added as a backdrop to provide a sharper focus and a means of identifying differences and similarities between complementary and conventional medical practices. "Energetic" or "mind/body" are terms used to describe an emergent energetic model of healing that encompasses in an interdependent mode physical, psychological, spiritual, social, and cultural perspectives. This energetic model is not new. It is traced to healing practices in ancient cultures like Greece, Egypt, India, and China, and is found in all periods of recorded history. In this study, the diverse practices represented in the energetic model share a view of the client as a total reality: body, mind, spirit. The four approaches employed by this energetic model--wellness, prevention, empowerment, and early intervention-- are shown to coincide with the central foci of the field of counselor education. As the emphasis in counseling and in other health care practices shifts toward preventive health and early intervention more attention will be focused on the need for greater client involvement and partnership between client and health care practitioner, the very cornerstones of complementary practices. The aim of these practices is to preserve and maintain a health that is not only the absence of disease, but rather, ideally, a "high-level wellness." Another aim is to provide meaning and purpose in all aspects of life, including the search for meaning and purpose in illness and disease, death, and dying; to empower clients and assist them with choices, hope, and relief of suffering. Finally the shifting of emphasis is from cure, which is an end-state and the ultimate goal of the conventional medical model, to healing as an evolving condition that can continue even unto death. The healing beliefs, approaches, and premises of complementary energetic practices, when studied individually, may appear quite insignificant as compared to those characterizing the large body of conventional medicine and psychotherapy. However, when taken collectively, they seem to form part of a jigsaw puzzle that is beginning to give shape to the formation of a new and more integrated view of reality. The findings from this study imply that counselor education programs could be enhanced by incorporating the techniques and approaches inherent in the energetic model. [Author Abstract]

21.) **Mauro, M. T.**

The effect of Reiki therapy on maternal anxiety
associated with amniocentesis.

M.N. thesis, University of Alberta (Canada). 2001.

The purpose of this pilot study was to determine

the acceptability and feasibility to conduct a

randomized controlled clinical trial to evaluate the

efficacy of Reiki therapy on the anxiety levels of

pregnant women about to experience their first

amniocentesis. Participants (n = 30) were

randomized to one of three groups (Reiki, Placebo,

Control). The anxiety levels of each participant

were assessed on seven occasions using the

Subjective Units of Disturbance Scale (SUDS), twice

using the Sheehan Patient Rated Anxiety Scale

(SPRAS), and once using an interview format. A total of 23 participants completed the study protocol. All participants reported significant differences in SUDS anxiety at different times throughout the amniocentesis. There was a differential treatment effect between the control group and both treatment groups immediately following the intervention. There was no difference in pre-treatment and post-treatment SPRAS scores. The feasibility and acceptability of conducting a larger study was supported. [Author Abstract]

22.)   McClenton, R.

Spirits of a lesser God: A critical examination of Reiki and Christ-centered healing.

Ph.D. dissertation, Trinity College and Seminary in Cooperation with the University of Liverpool (United Kingdom). 2006.

Reiki is an emerging adjunctive therapy that claims to provide physical and psychological healing as well as an experience of spiritual connection. It is increasingly employed in counseling centers, hospitals, and even churches. Reiki is believed by many to be a safe, non-invasive healing intervention that draws individuals towards God. Reiki practitioners maintain that they imitate Jesus' laying on of hands and claim that their praxis is the essentially the same as the healing used by Jesus as well as by Buddha. An ethnographic multi-case study was performed comparing the experiences of nine individuals, four who received Reiki therapy and five who received Christ-based hands-on healing. The long interview format was employed. The transcribed data were coded and analyzed for similar and distinct themes. In addition, a brief survey was utilized to determine the spiritual interests and involvement of each participant and the spiritual consequences of their healing experiences. The findings indicate that Reiki healing is distinct from that which is depicted in the Bible. Reiki appears to open up individuals to an "energy-based" healing modality that is spiritual in nature but is not specifically Christian. As reported by Reiki practitioners, it is a spirituality which welcomes shamanism, psychic healing, clairvoyance, spirit guides, and a host of other metaphysical practices as individuals become more intimately involved. In addition, the research demonstrates that Reiki therapy, over time, can cause physical, emotional, and spiritual harm. The writer contends that biblical healing, which at its core is soteriological and dependent upon the ministry of the Holy Spirit, heals mind, body, and spirit without harmful consequences. [Author Abstract]

23.)   **McGoldrick, J. R.**

Healers and the emerging healing profession: What are the implications for the practice of psychotherapy? Psy.D. dissertation, Argosy University/Orange County. 2002.

Although the art of healing dates back to ancient times, in the last three decades it has evolved into both a scientific practice and a viable profession. Variously known by such names as spiritual healing, energy healing, psychoenergetic healing, psychic healing, mental healing, and now, more commonly, simply "healing," the field now has attracted practitioners in the United States estimated to number from 15,000 to perhaps 500,000 or more. This Clinical Research Project reviews representative healing literature and reports the findings of a pilot qualitative study of four licensed clinical psychologists who integrate healing practices with traditional psychotherapy. The author examines the theoretical basis of healing--the existence of a field of unseen energy. Now most commonly called "subtle energy," this energy is thought to exist around and within the human body and is generally conceived of as higher levels of vibrations beyond normal perceptual abilities. She reviews efficacy studies of Therapeutic Touch, Reiki, and related forms of healing in the treatment of anxiety and stress and the enhancement of psychological well-being. Although she finds the research to be generally flawed, she concludes that the numbers of positive and mixed positive results suggest that a positive phenomena is likely at work. The author reports on commonalities among subjects in attitude toward the field of psychology, theoretical foundations, and phenomenological experiences of healing. Additionally, the range of subjects' approaches to integrating healing and psychotherapy are detailed as models for examining the implications of healing on the practice of psychotherapy. Questions addressed are those of ethics and legality, with attention to concerns regarding the use of touch in psychotherapy, scope of practice, and standard of care. [Author Abstract]

24.)   **Mitchell, K. C.**

Patients' and practitioners' experiences, perceptions and beliefs pertaining to the use of Reiki in dealing with chronic illness.

M.S. thesis, University of Saskatchewan (Canada). 2006.

Objectives: This qualitative study explored the experiences of patients suffering from cancer and other chronic conditions and those of their practitioners during a Reiki treatment. Specific research objectives were to: 1) better understand how participants describe healing, 2) document consecutive therapeutic encounters (i.e. Reiki sessions) as experienced by patients and practitioners over time and, 3) identify meaningful benefits and other relevant outcomes from both perspectives. Materials and Methods p*A convenience sample of four patient-practitioner pairs consented to participate in the study. Data was collected over 12 months via interviews with both the patients and Reiki practitioners. Hour long interviews were conducted before and after their participation in the study. Ten minute telephone interviews were done no longer than 48 hours after each Reiki session to capture participants' experiences with that particular session. All interviews were audio taped and transcribed. A phenomenological approach was used for the data analysis. Findings This qualitative study attempted to longitudinally explore the experiences and practices of Reiki from both the patients' and the practitioners' perspectives. Illness specific symptom relief as well as mental and emotional effects such as decreased anxiety and a better ability to handle stressful situation were experienced by the patients. Spiritual awakening and connection was attributed to the Reiki sessions and the relationship established with their practitioner. Energy directed releases during the Reiki sessions were quite common. Some practitioners experienced different sensory experiences that they attributed to the Reiki energy. The experiences ranged from feeling the energy, temperature changes to seeing different objects during the Reiki treatment. Many of the experiences described by the participants support what has been written in the literature. However, certain concepts such as the evolving concept of healing as well as the altered perception of illness are newer concepts which are beginning to surface. Conclusion Patients' and practitioners' experiences helped to gain insight in to the therapeutic relationship and their evolving definitions of healing. Several outcomes were noted on the physical, mental and emotional levels of all participants. This information will help lay the groundwork for future research on Complementary therapies including Reiki. Acknowledgement The Department of Community Health and Epidemiology Devolved Scholarship Fund

University of Saskatchewan and Hope Cancer Help

Centre, Saskatoon Saskatchewan supplied funding.

[Author Abstract]

25.)   **Mulholland, P. J. A.**

Reiki and the Roman Catholic tradition: an
anthropological study of changing religious forms in
modern Ireland.

Ph.D. dissertation, National University of Ireland,
Maynooth (Ireland). 2006.

This thesis takes the practice of Reiki healing as a

case study of the emergence and appeal of New

Age beliefs and practices in Ireland. I chart the

emergence of new forms of religiosity in Ireland in

the second half of the 20th century and discuss the

religio-cultural history and socio-economic and

political circumstances in which they flourished.

Then, on the basis of a meticulous study of a Reiki

initiation workshop and the personal narratives of

participants, I argue that both the New Age

Movement and magical-devolutional forms of Catholicism are manifestations of unresolved emotional needs and cognitive predispositions stemming from early childhood experiences. I explain the preference for the heterodox New Age form of religiosity as being a product of crucial differences in the manner in which traditional religious representations were propagated and exemplified. And I argue that it was the confluence of a combination of distressing political and socio-economic circumstances that made the magico-religious, millenarian and miraculous claims of a relatively small section of the Irish population credible amongst a wider audience. [Author Abstract]

26.)   **Novoa, M. P.**
The effects of Reiki treatment on mental health professionals who are at risk for secondary traumatic stress.
Ph.D. dissertation, Louisiana State University. 2011.

The purpose of this cross-sectional experimental study was to examine the effects of Reiki on risk level for secondary traumatic stress (STS) among mental health professionals, such as, social workers and licensed professional counselor (LPCs). The sample (N=67) was mostly composed of master social work students (MSW) (61%) from the School of Social Work at Louisiana State University (LSU), professionals social workers (34%), and LPCs (5%). Study participants were randomly assigned to one of three treatment groups: Reiki, placebo or control group. Dependent variables measured at pretest and posttest were: risk level for STS, anxiety, depression, somatic symptoms, anger and hopelessness. Multivariate analysis of variance was conducted to determine if there was a difference between treatment groups. No significant difference was found between the Reiki, placebo or control groups on any of the variables measured. Implications for the social work profession are discussed. [Author Abstract]

27.)   **Ocker, D.**

Massage therapy: Is it just for the body?

Ph.D. dissertation, The Union Institute. 2004.

The purpose of this study was to examine the question, How does a massage therapist assist clients in dealing with emotional release occurring during bodywork? It involved three sub hypothesis questions: (1)What does a massage therapist need to know about clients to effectively treat them (i.e. medications, surgeries, outside environmental issues)? (2) What does a massage therapist need to do to create a safe environment for the client? (3)How do physical symptoms reported by the client manifest themselves from emotional problems? Research was based on participatory observation with seven case studies of individuals who sought massage therapy to assist with physical and/or emotional problems. After discussion between massage therapist and client(s) of several types of massage and related therapies, permission was granted to proceed. Therapies employed in this study included Swedish massage, trigger point therapy, Reiki, polarity, and craniosacral therapy. Results of this study included observed physical and/or emotional changes for each case study, efficacy of therapies chosen, subjective evaluations of clients, and suggestions for possible further studies. [Author Abstract]

28.)   **Plodek, J. L.**
The effects of daily Usui Ryoho Reiki self-treatment on
the perceived stress of staff nurses.
Ph.D. dissertation, Saybrook University. 2011.

Stress and stress-related diseases have reached
epidemic proportions in contemporary society, yet
there is little research on how self-care methods
might be used to reduce the work-related stress of
nurses. The purpose of this study was to evaluate
the effectiveness of using daily Usui Ryoho Reiki
self-treatments as self-care to reduce perceived
stress among nurses. The research was guided by
two hypotheses: (a) daily use of Usui Ryoho Reiki
would reduce cortisol levels, and (b) daily use of
Usui Ryoho Reiki would reduce the perceived level

of stress. This study used a mixed-method approach consisting of an experimental group (n = 11) and a wait=list control group (n = 11) for a total of 22 subjects. The mixed-method design included a randomized control trial, and utilized the Perceived Stress Scale, salivary cortisol samples, and daily practice logs, along with qualitative focus group interviews, with nurses using Usui Ryoho Reiki as self-care and with a control group. The sample size was smaller than planned and extraneous variables made continued participation in the study difficult. As a result, the findings of this study are inconclusive. The quantitative findings did not support the hypotheses; however, the qualitative focus groups findings evidenced a decrease in perceived stress, an increase in relaxation, and a decrease in physical symptoms such as palpitations. The marginal trending revealed in the results of the Perceived Stress Scale and cortisol testing, along with the focus group data, supports the need for further research. Research using a larger group sample over an extended period of time has the potential to determine whether Usui Ryoho Reiki for self-treatment is an effective self-care intervention, reducing stress among nurses.

[Author Abstract]

29.) **Prone, D. J.**

A study of the effects of learning and practicing The Radiance Technique ™ (authentic Reiki™) on the quality of life of people living with type 2 diabetes and on long-term practitioners.
Ph.D. dissertation, Institute of Transpersonal Psychology. 2002.

This study examined the effects of learning and practicing The Radiance Technique(TRT) on the quality of life of people living with Type 2 diabetes and long-term practitioners. In Part One, 22 people with Type 2 Diabetes attended a 2-day workshop during which they were instructed in the First Degree of TRT, followed by 8 weekly practice/support meetings. Quantitative and qualitative data were collected pre- and post-intervention. Nineteen people completed the program (California residents, 16 female, 3 male, 14 Caucasian, 2 African American, 2 Hispanic, and 1 West Indian). Quality of life was measured using: Profile of Mood States (POMS), State Trait Anxiety Index (STAI), Spirituality Assessment Scale (SAS), and Diabetic Quality of Life Scale (DQOL). Hemoglobin A1C levels were collected for 14 participants. Qualitative data were collected from the weekly support meetings and by interviews with 6 post-intervention participants. Participants showed significant improvement in quality of life (within subject MANOVA, $F_{[4, 14]} = 8.82$, $p = .001$). Changes in Hemoglobin A1C (-0.32%, +4.5%) showed an improving trend ($p = .056$) with a medium effect size ($r = .43$). Qualitative data supported these results, with participants reporting benefits including improved health, greater self-confidence and esteem, and a more positive outlook on life. Significant improvements were shown on all instruments (p = .001, .013, .39, and .003, respectively) and medium and large effect sizes (r = .66, .56, .48, and .64, respectively). Part Two investigated whether long-term practice of TRT was associated with positive change. Sixty-four experienced practitioners completed a personal profile and the Omega Life Change Inventory. Multiple regression analysis indicated that intensity of practice was the only significant predictor of change. Neophyte practitioners in Part One showed a trend towards similar changes after 3 months.

Results indicate that TRT may be an effective intervention in improving quality of life of a population with Type 2 diabetes. [Author Abstract]

30.)   **Ring, M. E.**
Reiki and changes in pattern manifestations: A Unitary Field Pattern Portrait research study.
Ph.D. dissertation, The Catholic University of America. 2006.

A qualitative study was conducted using the Science of Unitary Human Beings (SUHB) to describe the changes in pattern manifestations of unitary human beings who receive Reiki, and present the theoretical understanding of these changes from the perspective of the SUHB. This study was ontologically, epistemologically, and methodologically consistent. Eleven participants, ages 13--65, who experienced Reiki from six Reiki Masters, were interviewed and described their experiences, perceptions, and expressions following a Reiki session. All interviews were audiotaped, transcribed and synthesized using the eight processes of the Unitary Field Pattern Portrait research method (UFPP) during an eight-month period. Four different processes of synthesis were utilized, uncovering 448 themes, which were synthesized into eight resonating themes to create an aesthetic portrait describing the experience of Reiki. The portrait was interpreted from the SUHB to create the theoretical construction of Reiki experiences as: knowingly participating in change to seek relief from the manifestations of dissonant field rhythmicities experienced as bearing the burden of hardship, distress, suffering, and sorrow: integrality perceived simultaneously as warm and cool, neutral and intense, dark ice, tingling, warm and thick liquid patterning; resonancy experienced as speeding up and slowing down rhythms; helicy experienced as a transitioning awareness unfolding into a pandimensional awareness of stillness of mind where past and future melt into the timeless now of a heightened awareness; and helicy unfolding as manifestations of continuously innovative, creative, diverse, unpredictable, and harmonious field rhythmicities, experienced as the all embracing embodiment of integrated awareness, harmony, and health. An increased sense of well-being and inner harmony are associated with maximum health. The information gained in this study supports Reiki as a method that enhances harmony and an increased sense of well-being. This research identifies new, nursing discipline specific knowledge by explicitly describing the transition from dissonance to harmony related to receiving Reiki, enriches nurses' understanding of the mutual human and environmental process, and lays the groundwork for the development of theory involving one way of actualizing human potentials that can enhance theory driven nursing practice. Further research is needed to investigate Reiki sessions given over time and in different populations. [Author Abstract]

31.)   **Segar, A. J.**

Exploring the concept of efficacy within complementary and alternative medicine: views of therapists and their patients.

Ph.D. dissertation, The University of Manchester (United Kingdom). 2009.

This study focuses on three CAM modalities, namely homeopathy, acupuncture and Reiki. These therapies have in common that they practice energy medicine and share elements of illness aetiology but are diverse in terms of training, methods and origins. Qualitative methods were used, primarily interviews undertaken in the North of England with 37 CAM therapists and 28 patients. In addition observation of therapy sessions, participation in therapy and correspondence and repeat interviews with key informants were carried out. The study found that, on one level, the efficacy of treatment can be understood in terms of symptom relief and a return to full health. This pragmatic notion of efficacy was in evidence here but only formed part of CAM therapists-patients understandings. Notions of efficacy are complex and nuanced based in part on interpretations of numerous signs. These interpretations may serve to instigate and reinforce conviction and belief in CAM efficacy. Furthermore ideas concerning energy medicine provide alternative models for health and the aetiology of illness. Understandings of efficacy are shaped by these models which serve to imbue illness with meaning and address a range of existential questions faced by those enduring suffering and affliction. Belief in CAM efficacy is often intimately intertwined with meanings and interpretations associated with CAM treatment and the personal qualities of CAM therapists. Understanding of CAM efficacy may involve all or some of the elements outlined above and can best be described as discursive and flexible involving elements spanning a spectrum from the practical and pragmatic to the esoteric and spiritual. [Author Abstract]

32.) **Sewduth, S.**

*The role of Reiki therapy in improving the quality of
life in people living with HIV.*

M.A. thesis, University of South Africa (South
Africa). 2008.

This qualitative study explored the use of Reiki in
improving the quality of life of people living with
HIV (PLWH). A purposive sample of seven
participants consented to the study. Reiki
attunement, self healing and data collection were
done over a six-month period. An idiographic
approach was used. The participants were
interviewed, then underwent Reiki attunement,
performed self healing for 21-30 days and were
interviewed again. Responses suggest that Reiki
therapy had positive outcomes. Illness-specific

symptom relief, increased levels of energy, improved sleeping patterns, decreased anxiety and depression, spiritual awakening and a better ability to handle stressful situations were reported. Reiki therapy enabled the participants to reappraise living with HIV, deal with anger, depression and self-blame. These positive changes led to some of them seeking employment, leaving destructive personal relationships and reconnecting with family members. The researcher strongly recommends further research in this area. [Author Abstract]

33.)   **Shore, A. L. G.**
The long-term effects of energetic healing on symptoms of psychological depression and self-perceived stress.
Ph.D. dissertation, Institute of Transpersonal Psychology. 2002.

Energetic or spiritual healing has been documented and practiced in nearly every civilization throughout the span of human existence (Benson, 1975). The present investigation examined the long-term effects of Reiki, a form of energetic healing, on symptoms of psychological depression and self-perceived stress as measured by the Beck Depression Inventory (BDI), Beck Hopelessness (HS), and Perceived Stress (PSS) scales. Fifty participants in need of healing were randomly assigned to one of three groups: hands-on Reiki

(Group 1), non-touch Reiki (Group 2), or Reiki placebo distance group (Group 3), and remained blind to treatment condition. Reiki practitioners provided participants with a free 1 1/2 hour treatment each week for a 6-week duration. Pretest data were collected before the onset of treatment; posttest data were collected upon completion of treatment 6 weeks later; and follow-up data were collected one year after completion of treatment. Repeated measures analyses, effect size computations, and Tukey post hoc comparisons assessed the long-term effects of hands-on, distance, and placebo distance Reiki treatments on symptoms of psychological depression and stress. Tests for change over time, correlations between measures, and qualitative data (interviews) provided additional analyses to further understanding of the experience and effects of energetic healing treatments. Findings demonstrated that although no significant difference between groups existed at pretest data collection, treatment groups exhibited significant reduction in depressive and stress symptomology as compared with controls. One year later, these findings were maintained. The results support research hypotheses of a significant long-term reduction of symptoms of depression (BDI), hopelessness (HS), and stress (PSS), exhibited by individuals in the treatment groups, as compared with control group participants at posttest and follow-up intervals. Findings demonstrate the therapeutic function of energetic healing on symptoms of psychological distress. The present investigation therefore recommends the integration of energetic healing into mainstream health care and traditional interventions. [Author Abstract]

34.) **Thornton, L. M.**

Effects of energetic healing on female nursing students.

M.S. thesis, California State University, Fresno. 1991.

An experiment was conducted to assess the effects of Reiki (an energetic healing modality), on anxiety, sense of personal power, and sense of well-being in female nursing students. The experimental group (N = 22) received a Reiki treatment from the trained Reiki practitioner. The control group (N = 20) received a Mimic-Reiki treatment from a research assistant who was trained in imitating a Reiki treatment. Instruments measuring anxiety (Spielberger State-Trait Anxiety Inventory) and personal power (Barrett Power as Knowing

Participation in Change Tool) were administered before and after treatment. A questionnaire assessed subjects' posttreatment sense of well-being. Hypotheses predicting that posttreatment Reiki subjects would report (a) significantly lower anxiety, (b) significantly greater sense of personal power, and (c) significantly greater sense of well-being than control subjects were not supported. Following treatment, State and Trait anxiety was significantly lower for both groups. [Author Abstract]

35.)   **Ventura Carraca, A.**
Reiki Treatment and Electroencephalographic
Correlations between Participants in Different
Locations.
M.A. thesis, Laurentian University (Canada).
2012.

Research on Reiki has been focused primarily on

the effects of Reiki treatments on physiology.

Previous studies have shown that Reiki can

produce certain changes on the recipient of a

treatment such has lower cortisol levels, lower

blood pressure and stabilizing heart rate, and also

decreased levels of depression, pain and anxiety.

The purpose of this study was to investigate the

electroencephalographic (EEG) profiles associated

with a Reiki treatment whether in a proximal

(Local) or distal (Non-Local) treatment where pairs of participants were separated by either a few centimetres or about 50 meters. Quantitative electroencephalography was used to record the simultaneous brain activity of pairs of Reiki practitioners and subjects or naïve volunteers engaging in Reiki procedures and subjects. Brain coherence showed increased theta power coherence for the Reiki pairs compared to sham pairs in the Non-Local and Local conditions. S_LORETA analyses demonstrated that Reiki pairs displayed greater shared activation within the frontal areas of the cerebrum whereas Sham pairs displayed more shared activation within the parietal regions. [Author Abstract]

36.)   **Vitale, A.**

Nurses' lived experience of Reiki for self-care.

Ph.D. dissertation, Villanova University. 2008.

The use of complementary and alternative
medicine (CAM) has increased over the years. In
recent years, there is a growing interest among
nurses, other health care providers and consumers
in CAM energy work that is non-invasive, not
dependent on technology, inexpensive, and holistic
in focus. Reiki is an energy-based healing practice
believed to have originated thousands of years ago
in the Tibetan Sutras and renewed in the 1800s by
Dr. Mikao Usui, a Japanese monk. Although the
inquiry about the usefulness of Reiki in patient care
has begun, there is little research to support the use

of Reiki touch therapy as a nursing intervention or as a self-care practice. The purpose of this study was to explore the lived experience of nurses who practice Reiki for self-care. A phenomenological approach was utilized to answer the research question, "What is the lived experience of nurses who practice Reiki for self-care?" In-person interviews were conducted with eleven nurses who met specific study criteria using open-ended questions to examine the experience of nurses who are Reiki practitioners, to understand their perceptions of Reiki use in self-treatment, and to appreciate its meaning for them. The Colaizzi method was utilized in data analysis and independent decision trail audits were completed to promote study rigor and trustworthiness of results. Thematic categories and major and minor thematic clusters emerged around the topics of daily stress management, self-healing, spirituality and interconnectedness of self, others and beyond. Implications of the study findings for nursing practice and nursing education are discussed. Potential applications of study findings to Jean Watson's transpersonal caring theory located within a caring science framework are explored and recommendations for future research are offered.

[Author Abstract]

37.) **Waldspurger Robb, W. J.**
The lived experience of registered nurse Reiki
practitioners: A phenomenologic study using
computer mediated communication.
D.N.Sc. dissertation, Widener University School
of Nursing. 2006.

The use of complementary and alternative

modalities (CAM) has increased over recent years

with healthcare consumers spending billions of

healthcare dollars on a variety of CAM therapies.

Reiki is an energy-based CAM therapy that is

derived from the ancient practices of Tibetan

monks. Proponents of Reiki believe that the

unblocking or redistribution of the body's natural

energy facilitates the body's ability to self-heal. The

purpose of this study was to describe the lived

experience of registered nurses who administer Reiki treatments to themselves and/or others. This study used computer-mediated communication to collect the research data from registered nurse Reiki practitioners from all levels of Reiki training. Interviews were conducted by electronic mail (email) using the Internet. Nineteen registered nurses who practice Reiki were interviewed via computer-mediated communication in order to answer the research question, "What is the lived experience of a registered nurse Reiki practitioner?". The purposive sample contained participants from 15 states representing a varied geographical area. Ricoeur's Interpretation Theory was utilized in data analysis. A preliminary model was constructed depicting the lived experience of registered nurse Reiki practitioners. This model contains four main parts, or wedges, each encompassing several themes, or sub-themes. Potential applications of Jean Watson's Theory of Human Caring and her Clinical Caritas and Conti-O'Hare's concept of Nurse as Wounded Healer for the Preliminary Model of the Lived Experience of the Registered Nurse Reiki Practitioner are presented. Methodological issues related to computer-mediated communication as a data collection methodology are revealed. Implications of the study findings on the discipline of nursing are discussed. Study limitations are shared and

recommendations for future research are suggested

by the researcher. [Author Abstract]

38.)   **Weir, S. G.**
Physiological changes and subjective experiences of Reiki healers.
M.A. thesis, The University of Regina (Canada). 2004.

Previous research in the area of alternative therapies in general, and Reiki (a form of hands-on healing) in particular, is limited. In the present study, the physiological changes and subjective experiences of healers during a Reiki healing session were examined to ascertain whether Reiki, as traditionally practiced, is correlated with measurable physiological changes in the body of the healer and to enhance knowledge of the healer's subjective experience. The participants included two groups: Reiki Master healers (n = 12) and mimic healers (n = 12), matched for age, education and sex. Differences were looked at for five measures (temperature, respiration rate, heart rate, skin conductance and EEG) before, during and after a healing session. It was hypothesized that, similar to the relaxation response, the healers would experience decreased brain wave activity, respiration rate, heart rate and skin conductance. The hypotheses was not supported. There were no significant differences between groups for these measures and no significant changes over time for these measures. It was also hypothesized that peripheral temperature would increase. Significant differences were found between groups for the measure of peripheral temperature. Repeated

Measures ANOVA indicated that there was a significant change in peripheral temperature for healers over time. The subjective experiences of the healers in this study included reports of many sensations (e.g., tingling, 'pins and needles', heat, coolness, shaking, pulsating, and swirling). Research in the areas of human energy fields, and of healers who treat energy fields, may encourage further studies. Studies could be carried out with other human energy field techniques (e.g., reflexology, acupuncture), with other cultural healers (e.g., shamans, healers from other countries), and with specific populations (e.g., those suffering from depression, anxiety, pain). More detailed healer profiles could be conducted to better understand individuals who work in this

area as well as more detailed profiles of individuals

who access alternative therapies and why they

choose these methods. [Author Abstract]

39.) **Winnegge, K. A.**

When East meets West an exploratory study of how Reiki is integrated into psychodynamic practice: a project based upon an independent investigation.
M.S.W. thesis, Smith College. 2011.

This study was undertaken to explore the experience of mental health professionals who use Reiki in their therapeutic practice. Secondly, the study examined clinicians' perceptions of the efficacy of Reiki in a mental health setting. Recruitment letters were sent out via internet professional listservs to individuals who held both Reiki certification and mental health licensure. Sixteen participants, twelve social workers and four licensed mental health counselors, were interviewed regarding their views on the integration of Reiki within their practice. Narrative data was collected that described clinicians' personal experiences with Reiki, their practice and how they considered Reiki as a therapeutic intervention within their profession. The findings of this study supported the previous literature that Reiki has been proven to alleviate tension and anxiety, decrease the perception of pain improve communication among clinician and client, and reduce emotional distress. Virtually all the clinicians in the sample noted that Reiki speeds up the therapeutic process for their clients as well as creating a body-mind awareness that may have been lacking before Reiki integration. Findings from this research may contribute to the ongoing dialogue regarding therapeutic touch and body-based clinical social work practice. As shifting trends indicate a need for an expanded approach to healing, including holistic medicine, the following research may convey an implication for expanded education in clinical social work practice. [Author Abstract]

40.)   **Woessner, E. M.**

The integration of energy work and psychotherapy.
Psy.D. dissertation, Massachusetts School of
Professional Psychology. 2007.

This dissertation examines the potential for the
integration of energy-based healing techniques
with traditional verbal psychotherapy. While
psychology has conceptualized the human being
according to a biopsychosocial model, energy
techniques seek to address the energetic or spiritual
level of human existence. The literature review
explores the history, techniques and current
practice of three hands-on energy healing
modalities: Reiki, Therapeutic Touch, and Healing
Touch. The available literature indicates that these

techniques may hold value in evoking the relaxation response, and primarily reports on their use within medical settings. The author interviews eight licensed psychotherapists of various professional identities, who also currently practice some energy techniques. The interviews were analyzed for similarities and differences among participants. Nine themes emerged from the analysis of the interviews, including: the energy paradigm as integrative or complementary versus alternative; the degree of explicit integration of energy techniques with verbal therapy; the role of the body as bridge to energetic awareness; pervasive contact with and awareness of the energetic level; seeking clients' higher self as a guide in treatment decisions; sources of therapists' guidance in treatment decisions; attributions of underlying causes of symptoms; the mechanisms of healing illness; and, the importance of peer supervision/collaboration. The results suggest a model for understanding the impact of life experiences on the energetic system and the mechanisms by which healing occurs on the energetic level. [Author Abstract]

41.) **Zephyr, L. H.**

The complementary function of touch during eidetic image therapy.

Ph.D. dissertation, Institute of Transpersonal Psychology. 1987.

This study investigates the use of touch to stimulate resolution of the conflicted psychic material brought into awareness through Eidetic Image Therapy. By touch is meant the laying of hands on the clothed body of the subject, with the individual's full acceptance that this contact facilitates a sense of safety and peace. The therapist is simply willing to ``be there'' and uses no form of mental invasion or persuasion. The foundation of this dissertation is Eidetic Image theory, research, and clinical techniques. The use of Reiki is an innovation of this process and shares with Eidetic Image Therapy the goal of the unification of mind, body, and emotional experience. The hypothesis was that the sense of emotional safety, physical relaxation, and personal experience of self that touch enhanced would help to dissolve the defense mechanisms and allow a new positive and unified experience. This hypothesis proved to be supported by clinical evidence. From 150 collected sessions, 7 single sessions and 1 case history are presented for analysis. These were chosen to show the varying individual responses during the image and Reiki touch portions of the therapy. Individual sessions are used to explicate the process, rather than case histories, to show the developmental progression of the subject. Indications of resolutions of conflict include the observations of changes in image content, body sensations, and emotional affect as reported by the subject and observed by the therapist. Findings indicate with remarkable consistency that touch creates positive physical and emotional change and this change is observed in modification of the image content. [Author Abstract]

Locating Dissertations and Theses

A. Purchase

Many of the dissertations and theses listed in this bibliography are available for purchase through UMI Dissertation Express:

http://disexpress.umi.com/dxweb

By Fax:

800-864-0019

By Mail:

789 E. Eisenhower Parkway, P.O. Box 1346, Ann Arbor, Michigan 48106-1346

800-521-3042

B. Interlibrary Loan

Dissertations and theses may also be requested through Interlibrary Loan via your local public, college or university library.

www.ingramcontent.com/pod-product-compliance
Lightning Source LLC
Chambersburg PA
CBHW070137290526
45789CB00002B/521